Your Guide to Assisted Living in Arizona

*What You Should Know Before
Placing Your Loved One*

Tammy and Russell Burns
With Cindy Abrams, RN, BS

Published by Wheatmark®
2030 East Speedway Blvd., Suite 106
Tucson, Arizona 85719 USA
www.wheatmark.com

ISBN: 978-1-60494-809-7 (paperback)
ISBN: 978-1-60494-845-5 (ebook)
LCCN: 2012941236

rev201201
rev202402

Contents

Foreword

Your Guide to Assisted Living in Arizona is a book that addresses issues unheard of just a few years ago. Planning for disability and incapacity is a relatively new phenomenon. While we have always known death to be inevitable, the likelihood of an extended period of time in which an individual requires assistance with personal care and activities of daily living was not part of the equation until the last fifty years or so.

In the United States, life expectancy in 1900 was just over 49 years. In 1950, life expectancy was about 68. Now, it is near 80 for most Americans. Beginning in 2011, 10,000 people turn 65 every day—a rate of growth that is expected to continue for almost 20 years. Many of these people will continue to live healthy and productive lives for years. Many, though, will need some degree of care.

Fifty or sixty years ago, even when people did need care prior to the end of life, that care was often provided by family members who would rally together to take care of their elderly and infirm. But as society changed in the mid twentieth century, family structure and demographics changed dramatically. Children moved away. Economic and cultural changes resulted in more two-income families, leaving no one home during the day to provide care for aging parents or grandparents.

I recall my grandfather's death in the early 1960s. He was 68 or 69. He worked every day in his own business. My grandmother had died within the year, after a very short illness—I believe she had pneumonia. Although my grandfather appeared quite healthy, his four children, all of whom had remained in the metropolitan Detroit area, expressed concern for his well-being after his wife's death. Each of the four children had a traditional family with one working spouse and one who stayed at home. The children and older grandchildren took turns staying at Papa's house each night so he wouldn't be alone. It was not long before he began complaining of respiratory symptoms himself. Remembering the experience with my grandmother's pneumonia, the children took him to the doctor quickly. It was not pneumonia. Papa had lung cancer that was described to be very advanced. His treatment options were limited. They tried chemotherapy, but the side effects were devastating. He spent what seemed like weeks in the hospital before his death.

Now, the outcome would probably be much different. Medical advances have provided many ways of extending life – sometimes with quality, sometimes without. Now, cancer would probably be diagnosed much earlier with the incredible diagnostic tools and technologies that were not available back then. My grandfather would have had a number of sophisticated treatment options and would have possibly lived a long time, with or without the cancer. Now, two-thirds of those diagnosed with cancer have a five-year or longer survival rate. That was certainly not the case back then.

Modern society is different, as Russell and Tammy Burns point out. Now, Papa may live long enough to experience a number of other impairments. He may develop dementia, as have one in seven Americans over 70. Maybe he would fall and break a hip. More than one-third of people over 65 fall each year—300,000 of them will fracture a hip. Chronic disorders and physical limitations increase greatly with advanced age. And, although there are still family caregivers, in many cases there is nobody. Children often live far away or are simply unable to provide the level of in-home assistance required. Retirees often leave the area where they raised their family and seek better climates and better economic conditions elsewhere. In too many cases, no family member is willing or able to provide the needed care.

This is why this book is so valuable. How can people assure adequate care for their loved ones or themselves? What are the processes, procedures, and protocols? Where do you go for help? How can families plan for the increasing likelihood that someone will need some level of long-term care at some time? How can they deal with these issues if, like so many, they did not plan for them? These are the questions addressed in *Your Guide to Assisted Living in Arizona* by Tammy and Russell Burns and Cindy Abrams. They speak from experience, as they have worked in these trenches for years. And they speak from the heart. Tammy and Russell have watched the need for long-term care grow and they have personally responded to that growing need with caring and loving attention. There are few people in Arizona who know this industry as well as Tammy and Russell. Here, in this short, well-organized book, they pass along their knowledge and experience with kindness, compassion, and sensitivity. Thank you, Tammy and Russell.

Ronald Zack, Attorney and Registered Nurse
Ronald Zack, PLC
Elder Care Law and Estate Planning

Preface

This book is the result of our learning the assisted living industry, both small homes and large centers, from the inside out. In Arizona, a center is a facility licensed for more than 10 people, and a home is licensed for 10 or fewer. Together we have over 40 years combined experience, both in centers and homes. During this time, we have learned our role in managing and caregiving, and have seen the frustrations families experience as they attempt to navigate the long-term care system. With this book, we hope to provide a tool for our own families and for others who will face the many decisions related to long-term care in the near future.

We have chosen to write from *us* to *you*. We are assuming that you are the one pursuing long-term care options for your loved one: Mom, Dad, Grandpa, Aunt Sally, etc., and we will use those terms interchangeably with resident.

We write from the point of view of assisted living center and home manager/owner. Our greatest experience caring for people is in a 10-bed home environment, although we interact regularly with larger facilities and with people in their own homes. We believe that for the majority of those requiring hands-on assistance, the assisted living home is by far the best alternative, and this book will primarily deal with that context. But there are times, especially if someone is very independent and high functioning, when a larger center is advantageous. Some of these advantages include:

- **Transportation.** Large centers generally provide a schedule of regular outings to various shopping locations around town (Kmart, Walmart, grocery stores, shopping malls), in addition to individual appointments. These may be charged separately.

- **Activities.** Large centers tend to have an extensive activity program. If this interests you, be sure to visit during those activities to see who participates and if it is, indeed, what you have in mind. Keep in mind, however, your loved one's preference for activities, rather than what you think he or she should do.

- **Dining.** Generally, restaurant-style dining is available, with various selections, rather than home-style cooking, where everyone eats basically the same menu.

- **Community.** There is a larger population in a center and therefore a greater likelihood of finding more people to whom your loved one can relate.

- **In-house services.** Often, the larger center will have an on-site hair salon, a gift shop, a rehab or exercise facility, and other services that might be of interest.

- **Medical services.** Most of the centers have a nurse on duty 40 or more hours per week. These nurses usually don't do actual nursing care, so please be sure to ask what their role is in the facility. This may vary, as many conditions are treated by Medicare-certified home health agencies, just as they are in smaller assisted living homes. If you would prefer a homey atmosphere, discuss this with the care home to find out exactly what they can and cannot do.

We hope you find this guide a simple and practical tool for gaining understanding of the major issues you face. We intentionally reduced the clutter of excessive information within the primary text; appendices at the end of the book contain useful forms, checklists, and instructions for navigating various aspects of the health-care system in Arizona. You also can access new and current information and FAQs on our website, www.integratedglobal.coach, at any time.

Introduction: Why You Need This Book

This guidebook is a must-have for everyone approaching the season of long-term care, whether it be for yourself or a loved one. You might be a doctor or an RN, a son or daughter, or a neighbor. You might be someone who knows a person approaching the need for long-term care, or you might be that person yourself. We hope you are planning ahead for what might be coming down the road. *Do not wait* until you need long-term care for a loved one. Research the options early and know what you will face, should the need arise.

This guide is designed to empower you, the consumer, so that you can make informed decisions about the long-term care system, while at the same time raising the standard of adult assisted living in your community. As you are informed and educated, the industry automatically will rise up to meet the higher standard demanded. This is our desire: the highest standard of care for those requiring it and your confidence in that care as you place your loved one. By understanding your options, you will be able to make the best decisions in situations that often are highly stressful.

⟿ KEY POINT ⟿

Our purpose is to help you understand the system and your role in it, to define reasonable expectations, and to give you the tools you need to secure the best care.

The Baby Boomers

What was once on the horizon is now upon us: the season called retirement and senior citizenship. In 2006, the first baby boomers turned 60, officially opening the floodgates. As with every season in the lives of this generation, the entire nation will shift in order to meet their demands. They needed diapers and baby food in the 1940s and 1950s; they needed fast food in the 1950s and 1960s. They participated in the housing boom in the 1970s and the credit craze in the 1980s and 1990s. Now, many have ushered their kids out into the world and are enjoying the empty nest.

Close on the horizon comes the season of Medicare, Social Security, and the ever-looming long-term care. Analysts have talked about this coming event for years. Will Medicare and Social Security hold up? We will soon see.

Regardless, this is what is and will continue to happen: a huge population will require all kinds of medical and daily-living assistance. In most cases, it will fall to their children to walk down this road with them. We have walked it with various people and are convinced a guidebook like this will not only be helpful but indispensible in the quest for excellent care for Mom and Dad.

The Nature of the Task

Almost all of us are novices in securing long-term care for a loved one. There generally are just a few people in our lives in this season of life—our parents, maybe an aunt or uncle, a grandparent, or a close friend—and not all of them require long-term care. When we start looking into care, we're uneducated, and when we finish, we may understand the system better than we'd like to understand it.

System Breakdown

The consumer (that's you) is largely at the mercy of the system, and that's a very scary place to be— the system is not designed to be helpful. Most people with whom you talk will know their own area of expertise and little else.

Furthermore, nearly every agency out there, regardless of what they tell you, represents someone who is making money by way of your loved one's care, and they will usually lead you into the arena that pays them the best. Most of the time they mean well, but it's big business, and unfortunately, too often it is designed with profit as the goal, not the best care for your loved one.

⟶ KEY POINT ⟶

Whether good or bad, the system is all we have. We hope to guide you through it, step by step, taking out some of the mystery and positioning you to make the best decisions regarding the care of your loved one.

If you have ever participated in the health-care system, whether through a brief stay in the hospital or an extended illness involving many practitioners, you know that the system is lacking, at best. Of course, within the system there are those who genuinely care and who are acutely interested in you and in your loved one's well-being. But the reality is that the system is filled with rules and regulations. On the surface, such rules seem designed to protect you, but in fact, oftentimes they are the result of endless lawsuits. The majority of rules are designed to protect the institutions. So we are left to navigate through a confusing web of bureaucracy in order to secure the assistance we need.

The health-care system is fragmented, with many individual entities providing specific services and under strict legal obligations to protect privacy. This inhibits the flow of communication from one branch of the system to another, and creates huge obstacles in the ability of the system to educate and support and to provide continuity of care.

As we have counseled many people through the process of caring for a loved one in the long-term care system, we have found a great many repeating scenarios. We will share fictional scenarios based on real-life experiences throughout the book. You may find stories similar to yours.

— 1 —

Be Proactive: Make a Plan Before the Need Arises

Grace's Story

It was a warm day in June when Grace woke early in the morning in her bedroom in the eastern suburbs of Tucson. At age 88, she had always been healthy and proud of her ability to care for herself and not be a burden to her family. She saw her doctor once or twice a year and took only a pill for her thyroid and a multivitamin each day. Her father had lived to be 97 and her mother 102. Grace had a number of good years left ahead of her, and she took good care of herself so that she could enjoy them independently. Her husband had passed away two years earlier. She missed him, but she kept herself busy and believed that she still had a purpose on earth.

As she sat up to head to the bathroom, she felt a bit dizzy. She had been feeling a little weak and under the weather over the past couple of days and thought maybe she had a touch of something that was going around. "Maybe I just need to drink more water," she thought. "That's probably it." She would make a point to do that, but then, of course, there would be the endless trips to the bathroom that came with drinking more water — and that seemed to be increasing these days and becoming more urgent, like now.

Grace stood up a little before she should have, and her legs just seemed to give out from under her. She stumbled and tried to catch her balance but to no avail. She crashed to the floor, toppling over a TV tray containing last night's dishes on her way down. Moments later, she opened her eyes. She wasn't sure if she had passed out and was waking up or if she had just fallen. She looked around and tried to move. That's when she became aware of an excruciating pain on her left side. She could not move without pain shooting everywhere and nearly causing her to lose consciousness.

She felt for the emergency call button she wore around her neck, but it wasn't there. She had taken it off last night in the shower and had forgotten to put it back on, which was very uncharacteristic of her. Everything seemed to spin inside her head from the pain and the confusion about what she should do. She tried calling out for help, but because she lived in a single-family house, she really didn't expect anyone to hear her. There was no phone within reach, and besides, her family had just left on vacation. She lay there in shock and pain, unsure of what to do next. She felt very frightened.

She wasn't sure how much time had passed when she woke up in the hospital. A woman was standing by her

bed, but Grace had no idea who she was. The woman re-
minded Grace that she was her neighbor, Lois. She had come
by Grace's house that afternoon with some nut bread, and
when Grace didn't answer the door, Lois suspected something might be wrong. She called 911. The paramedics found
Grace unconscious on the floor and brought her to the emergency room. Grace had no idea why she was found on the
floor. She tried to get up, but she was hooked up to all kinds
of machines. She asked for her husband, demanding that he
be notified right away. Lois explained to the doctor that this
was not like Grace—she was almost never confused.

When Lois was asked if anyone was designated to make
decisions on Grace's behalf, Lois was unable to answer.
Lois explained that Grace's daughter was out of town on
vacation—she had called her and was waiting to hear back.
Meanwhile, Grace explained that her daughter would be of
no use in this situation because she was only a child. She
again insisted that they must contact her husband.

Suddenly, Lois's cell phone rang. It was Grace's
daughter who said she would come right away, but it
would probably be a day before she and her family could
make it back. The daughter asked to speak with the medical
team at the hospital but was told that they could not share
anything about the patient's condition because they had no
written or verbal permission to do so.

This story brings up many issues of which people may be unaware, from health risks to interfacing
with the medical system to the question of who will
make decisions for Grace if she doesn't recover her
faculties. Many of Grace's problems could have been

avoided, but they also could have been much more complicated. Grace suffered from a urinary tract infection (UTI). A UTI can come on quickly and cause a perfectly sane person to become forgetful and confused, almost overnight. It also causes weakness and a need to urinate frequently. In the elderly, a UTI may go unrecognized, as it is not always accompanied by discomfort.

Because Grace was the picture of health, she hadn't made plans for someone to have her medical power of attorney in the event that she should become unable to make decisions herself. Grace was at the mercy of the system, which is designed to make money and protect itself from lawsuits first and to do its best for the patient second.

In Grace's case, the doctors ran tests, discovered the UTI, and put her on antibiotics. The fall caused a broken hip that would require surgery. By the time the family arrived the following morning, Grace was back to her sharp self and was able to give consent for the family to make decisions on her behalf. Suddenly, the family was placed in the overwhelming position of taking care of Mom, who very likely would not be able to return home and live alone again.

Obtain Necessary Documents Early

Grace's story is a classic example of the need for everyone to have some plan or to think about long-term care solutions for their loved ones much earlier than may seem necessary. In Grace's case, the need was sudden and obvious. Often, it is not so clear. We cannot stress enough the importance of establishing your plans and legal authority to represent your loved one as early as possible. And it is never too early.

⟶ KEY POINT ⟶

A parent often feels threatened by his or her children moving into a parenting role. Discussing these matters before any signs of decline present themselves can radically reduce conflict. Both parties can plan for the inevitable before the inevitable bears down on them.

Medical and Financial Powers of Attorney

It's never too early for emergency planning, but it can quickly become too late. Seniors often are reluctant to give their children power of attorney because they fear losing control over their lives. However, a power of attorney is only applicable when a person is incapable of making decisions. It's important to reinforce that the best way for seniors to control their future care needs is to plan for them when they're not in a crisis situation. Furthermore, having all the appropriate documents, allowing for health care and other decisions before they are needed for long-term care, will save hundreds and maybe thousands of dollars, not to mention endless stress, time, and hassle. Trying to obtain control over Dad's resources after he has become confused and untrusting requires a long, painful, and costly journey through the legal system. Consider the following story.

Jim's Story

Jim, 87 years old, had lived alone in his home in Scottsdale ever since his wife, Margaret, passed away. She had had a very slow-progressing form of cancer, and Jim had cared for her meticulously during the last five years of her life. They had hired a housekeeper some 10 years before her passing, and this housekeeper, Patricia, had gradually become somewhat of a caregiver, assisting Jim in the care of his wife. Patricia was a very hard worker and was extremely devoted to Margaret and Jim.

Jim had very high standards and an extremely high level of compassion. After Margaret died, Jim felt that it made sense to have Patricia move in and become a full-time housekeeper/caregiver for him, as there were many things with which he was beginning to need assistance, and he didn't think he should be home alone. He had two children—a daughter, Monica, in Flagstaff, and a son, Mike, in Florida. Although they called and visited from time to time, they never really interfered with their dad's life, and he never asked them for help.

While visiting one Thanksgiving, Mike watched while his dad signed a check that Patricia had filled out. Jim said it was Patricia's paycheck, and she now was helping him manage his financial affairs. This concerned Mike, so he *began to look into things a bit. Mike noticed that his dad's short-term memory was beginning to slip—he would frequently forget things he had said or done.*

It turned out that Patricia was collecting three and sometimes four $750 checks per week, to the tune of $10,000 to $15,000 per month. When Mike confronted his dad about this, he was met with a severe rebuke and was told to mind his own business. Jim had become completely dependent on Patricia to care for him.

Jim trusted Patricia and was unwilling to part with her, even when confronted with her gross mismanagement and theft. He would admit that she was not perfect, but he would do nothing to jeopardize his relationship with her.

Mike went to his lawyer to find out how to gain some say in his dad's life, for his own good, but he found it to be extremely difficult. His dad would have to sign a release or authorize his son to act as his power of attorney, or Jim would have to be deemed incompetent by a court, which was a very expensive and slow process. Jim was a stubborn man and would not have anyone running his life. Because he already perceived his children as trying to interfere with what he knew he wanted, he refused to sign any documents. Mike went to the authorities with all the evidence he had, but they said that as long as Jim was competent and willingly signing checks, there was nothing they could do.

Mike and Monica wanted to respect their dad's wishes, so, unsure what to do, they stood back and watched while his caregiver drained his accounts. One day, Patricia's paycheck bounced. A week later, Mike received a phone call from his dad. Patricia had vanished. Jim was devastated and now had no funds to provide for his care.

This story, although fictional, has played itself out in many lives and will continue to do so, as long as people don't understand the laws that govern aging adults. Some families stand back and let Dad run his own life, while others choose to intervene, go down the very painful road of conflict, and feel guilty for stripping Dad of his independence. Neither option is pleasant. What follows are some safeguards you can put in place to help protect your loved one before it's too late.

Know What's Going on in Dad's Life

You should know who's who in the lives of your loved ones. Meet and talk regularly with their banker, accountant, lawyer, doctors, friends, neighbors, and anyone else who is in regular contact with them. This is especially important if you live far away and don't see them on a regular basis. If you are far away, you may want to consider a nurse advocate or case manager to help you stay on top of the situation.

Be alert for changes that could signal the beginning of a decline. As you evaluate your aging family member's ability to continue living at home without assistance, look for the following signs, as problems in one or more of these areas may call for further assessment and possibly part-time help in the home, such as housekeeping, meal services, or medication management:

- **Short-term memory loss:** forgetting to take medication, appointments, meals, bathing

- **Fall risk:** balance problems, frequent falls, general unsteadiness

- **Difficulty managing personal care:** bathing, eating, toileting, personal hygiene (activities of daily living, known as ADLs)

- **Financial mismanagement:** unpaid bills, overpaid bills, unawareness of current financial situation

- **Trouble getting around:** loss of ability to drive safely or secure other means of transportation

- **Weight loss or gain:** inability to prepare meals and obtain proper nutrition

- **Isolation:** inability to use a telephone

- **Poor judgment:** obsession about spending money, not eating wisely, fear of leaving the home, being too trusting or too suspicious of others

Medical, Financial, and Personal Affairs

Planning for unforeseen health-care emergencies is something everyone should do, regardless of age. Of course, the older we get, the more of an issue this becomes. If your loved one begins to have health concerns, get into a position, as soon as possible, where you can take control legally of your loved one's finances, should the need arise. Again, the issue of trust here is huge. Even the closest and most loving families can develop weird feelings when someone perceives a threat to money and control. It is a good idea to have a trusted family friend, accountant, or lawyer involved in conversations as you work through this. Often, a third party with no emotional investment can help bridge the gap when emotions of those involved are running high. There are many options available, including a trust or conservatorship, which passes financial decision making to a neutral party.

It is strongly suggested that you discuss these matters in detail with your attorney or CPA. You must understand the laws governing what you can and cannot do, and you must act with integrity so that you don't inadvertently take what isn't yours. Below are common structures that provide the access you need:

Power of attorney is the authorization to act on someone else's behalf in a legal or business matter. The person authorizing the other to act is the *principal, grantor,* or *donor,* and the person authorized to act is the *agent, proxy,* or *attorney-in-fact.* It's important to note that a power of attorney of any type is only valid when the principal is physically or mentally incapable of making decisions (there must be documentation supporting this) or when the principal chooses to activate it. The law requires the agent to be completely honest with and loyal to the principal in their dealings. There are various types of powers of attorney. For example, a health-care power of attorney empowers the proxy to make medical decisions on the principal's behalf. Other powers may be limited to circumstances in which the grantor is incapacitated. It is best to discuss these issues with an attorney who can guide you in what will best suit your situation.

Advance directives or living wills are written statements that define someone's wishes for medical care, in the event that person is rendered unable to communicate. This may be general or very detailed. It may or may not identify people who will make decisions for the person. We recommend obtaining an advance directive as soon as possible. Either you or a trusted friend or family member should have a copy so that if Mom becomes unable to make decisions, her wishes will be known, and you can legally direct the doctors. Physicians carry a huge liability and are governed by many laws that specify to whom they can talk. They have the right to refuse to work with even a well-meaning family member who has no legal authority to direct the care of his or her loved one. Arizona has a program through the Attorney General's office in which anyone can register his or her advance directives so that health-care workers can access them as needed.

Orange Cards are papers or small cards that tell paramedics what someone wants done should the person's heart or breathing stop. In Arizona, health-care workers can honor advance directives and living wills, but *paramedics cannot*; they follow instructions on the Orange Card. If it would be your choice *not* to have CPR or advanced life support should your heart or breathing stop, you should have an Orange Card. It's called an Orange Card because the instructions must be printed on bright orange paper to be valid. Many physicians' offices have these available, or you can obtain them from the Arizona Attorney General's office.

Resources. One extremely valuable resource to help cover all bases regarding medical directives and living wills is a booklet called *The Five Wishes*, available free at www.integratedglobal.coach. This booklet is for anyone of any age. Whether completing it for yourself or your loved one, it will help you determine who you want to make decisions for you, should you lose the ability to do so. It also specifies advance medical directives stating your wishes for the end of life. It is simple and yet thorough, and in Arizona, all authorities respect it at the same level as any legal document. You also can download a Life Care Planning Packet from the Attorney General's website, azag.gov, or request that one be sent to you by calling 800-352-8431. The power of attorney and primary care physician must have a copy of any advance directives or living wills.

Emergency contact numbers. Keep these in convenient places. We recommend printing such numbers on a small card and carrying it with you (and have your parent do so too). Put the card in a wallet or your car's glove box in case of an emergency while out alone. Accidents, strokes, and heart attacks can come out of nowhere and leave a person immediately unable to give the simplest directions.

Health information. It's important to keep a list of all diagnoses, allergies, and medications that easily can be given to emergency room or urgent care staff, should the need arise. Remember to revisit this list every few months to make sure it's current. It's a good idea to also keep this information in your loved one's purse or wallet.

Funeral arrangements and burial plans. These are much easier to talk about and work through when nobody is dying. Take the time to plan while you are not under the stress of losing or having just lost a loved one. As you approach the subject of caring for your loved ones when they can no longer care for themselves, you must talk, talk, and talk. Talk while you still can.

Long-Term Care Options

Today's long-term care options are endless. The best approach is to develop a strategy and have a plan ready, should the need for long-term care arise.

Shop around and know what the options are in your area. Keep a notebook or journal of places you visited or companies you talked to, so you'll remember which ones you liked. (It's hard to remember these details when you're in a crisis situation.) When possible, take Mom and Dad with you. Search the Department of Health Services (DHS) website (azdhs.gov/als/) and learn about homes within your ZIP code. Visit some nursing facilities and make notes of your impressions. Interview home-care providers, and investigate nurse advocacy or case management services available in your area. You will be much more objective if you create a plan in advance than if you search under the pressure of having to place or find care for Mom or Dad immediately.

⟿ KEY POINT ⟿

Remember: As you approach the subject of caring for your loved ones when they can no longer care for themselves, you must talk, talk, and talk. Talk while you still can.

Discuss what would be important to your loved ones if they had to move into long-term care. Cover various scenarios: stroke, hearing loss, vision loss, loss of ability to walk, loss of mental capacity. What would they want in each situation? Nothing is set in stone, but understanding what quality of life looks like from their point of view will take a lot of the mystery out of your decisions when the time comes. In the next chapter, we will look at the various options for long-term care and define many of the terms you will encounter.

— 2 —

Long-Term Care Overview

The terms *assisted living, long-term care,* and *skilled nursing* are often used interchangeably, but they are different. As you move into this realm, it's helpful to have a good command of a few important terms. These definitions are taken from AZ Statutes: Title 9–Chapter 10–Article 7-701, definitions that can be found online at www.integratedglobal.coach or under "Arizona Administrative Code" at www.azdhs. gov/als/hcb/index.htm.

Long-Term Care Options

Independent living applies to apartment-style facilities in which elderly residents can mostly care for themselves, but because of the frailty that comes with aging, wish to be in a more secure environment. Usually, services include meals (available in a dining room), weekly housekeeping, activities, and transportation. Individuals are responsible for their laundry, personal care, and medications.

Assisted living applies to senior living facilities that provide care in addition to housing, meals, and activities. In Arizona, assisted living is defined as a *residential care institution, including adult foster care, that provides or contracts to provide supervisory care services, personal care services, or directed care services on a continuing basis.* These facilities are either homes (10 or fewer residents) or centers (11 or more residents). They cannot perform ongoing nursing activities, such as maintaining IVs. In many instances, services can be provided by a home health agency in an assisted living facility, if the patient doesn't require 24-hour nursing supervision.

Medicare-certified home health agencies provide some intermittent nursing services, such as short-term daily injections, wound care, diabetes education and training, or monthly catheter changes in assisted living facilities. They also can provide physical, occupational, and speech therapy two to three times a week in the facility. There is no fee or co-pay for Medicare home health services, and they can continue as long as the person qualifies for services under Medicare guidelines. Many assisted living residents may qualify for hospice care within the facility. Medicare's hospice benefit also has no fee or co-pay.

Hospice services are a Medicare benefit that can provide care in assisted living facilities. Hospice is specialized care designed for those who have an illness that could shorten their lifespan to less than six months. The hospice will send in a nurse one or more times a week, as well as provide other services to help support not only the patient but his loved ones as well on the end-of-life journey. Hospice also will completely cover incontinence supplies, oxygen, most medical equipment, and some medications. With this type of added care, most assisted living facilities generally can care for residents all the way through hospice.

Skilled nursing applies to facilities also known as nursing care institutions or nursing homes. They are health-care institutions that provide inpatient beds and nursing services to persons who need this type of care on a continuing basis but who do not require hospital care or direct daily care from a physician. These facilities can care for all levels of physical and cognitive decline. They also have either an RN or LPN on duty at all times.

Assisted Living Levels of Care

Within assisted living, there are various levels of care for which specific rules and regulations apply. *Applicable statutes are quoted in italics.*

Supervisory care services *means general supervision, including daily awareness of resident functioning and continuing needs, the ability to intervene in a crisis, and assistance in the self-administration of prescribed medications.* This level is limited to supervision without hands-on assistance. Administering medications is not permitted at this level, and neither is caring for a confused person who is unable to self-direct.

Personal care services *means assistance with activities of daily living that can be performed by persons without professional skills or professional training and includes the coordination or provision of intermittent nursing services and the administration of medications and treatments by a nurse who is licensed pursuant to Title 32, Chapter 15, or as otherwise provided by law.* This basically refers to all levels of nonmedical physical assistance and assistance taking medications.

Directed care services *means programs and services, including supervisory and personal care services, provided to persons who are incapable of recognizing danger, summoning assistance, expressing need, or making basic care decisions.* This category accounts for dementia and cognitive disabilities. It is the most comprehensive care.

Who's Caring for Your Loved One?

A number of different levels of trained staff will care for your loved one. Most people who require 24/7 care do not need an entire skilled nursing staff, which comes with a very high price tag. Instead, in assisted living situations, what a person needs most is the presence of people who can help with daily living activities and who can recognize issues that may need attention. The following are some of the professionals who serve in assisted living facilities:

Certified caregivers. Arizona requires all caregivers working in assisted living facilities to complete a state-approved training program. Caregivers are certified at three levels, which correspond to the care levels defined above (supervisory, personal, and directed). Caregivers are trained in assisting with activities of daily living, laundry, nutrition, meal preparation, giving medications, and recognizing signs of when to call in the doctor. A certified caregiver must be at least 18 years old. Anyone left alone with patients must be at least 21 years old and certified at all the home's levels of care. In addition, they must supply proof of freedom from tuberculosis on an annual basis and keep their CPR and first-aid training updated. They must have a fingerprint clearance card on record.

Assistant caregivers. They can help a certified caregiver or manager with care but only when a certified caregiver or manager is physically present. They must be at least 16 years old, but they must be at least 18 years old to help with bathing, toileting, transfers, medications, or treatments. Assistant caregivers must also meet the same fingerprint, tuberculosis testing, CPR, and first-aid requirements as a caregiver.

Certified nursing assistants (CNA). They have completed a state- approved nursing assistant program, taken a state-issued exam, and received a certificate issued by the state board of nursing. To work in assisted living, they also must complete additional training mandated by the Department of Health Services (DHS). They are regulated by both the board of nursing and DHS. A CNA must meet the same requirements as a certified caregiver and will have the same duties.

Licensed managers. Managers of assisted living

facilities are licensed by the Arizona Board of Examiners of Nursing Care Institution Administrators and Assisted Living Facility Managers, following successful completion of a state-issued exam. They have a good understanding of the laws that govern the industry, a working knowledge of the nursing skills they manage on a daily basis, and skills in working with people. To become managers, they must work in the health-care field full time for one year (or equivalent hours) and complete the state-mandated caregiver training. In addition, they must complete state-required manager's training. Managers are generally on call 24/7 and deserve a great deal of respect for the enormous responsibility they bear.

Licensed practical nurses (LPN). These are nurses trained in routine nursing care, who are allowed to perform complex tasks under the direction of a physician or registered nurse. LPNs are licensed by the Arizona State Board of Nursing.

Registered nurses (RN). An RN must complete a state-approved education program and pass an exam. RNs then are licensed by the state board of nursing.

Nurse practitioners (NP). A nurse practioner is an RN who has had additional training and is able to take on many activities normally carried out by a physician, such as diagnosing, ordering lab work or tests, and prescribing medications and treatments. NPs play a very valuable role in assisted living situations, as these practitioners are very hands-on and up-to-date on the issues facing the aging population.

Furthermore, because their entire clientele is generally elderly or homebound, they make house calls.

➤ KEY POINT ➤

Remember: In assisted living, what a person needs most is someone who can help with daily activities and who can recognize issues that need attention.

Who Pays for Assisted Living Care?

Assisted living is considered residential care, as opposed to medical care, per state regulations. Because of this, it is a "private pay" industry, which means your loved one must pay out of pocket for it. Although Medicare will cover home health or hospice services provided in the assisted living facility, it will not pay for assisted living itself.

Long-term care insurance. This type of policy may cover most assisted living facilities. If your loved one has this type of insurance, it's important to know what the policy covers and if there are any restrictions on the type of facility you choose. Some of these policies require that the assisted living facility have a nurse on call, on staff, or on duty at all times. In addition, there are policies that only will cover facilities licensed for 10 residents or more. Most of these policies will only pay for assisted living if the person needs hands-on assistance with at least two activities of daily living (ADLs). Meal preparation and medication management don't count as ADLs, so not everyone who needs to go to assisted living will meet these requirements when they first move in. The good news is they probably will qualify when their care needs increase.

Veterans Aid and Attendance. Veterans and their spouses (or widows) may qualify for benefits to assist with the cost of care under this program. This program pays the person who qualifies directly, and then that person can choose how to spend the funds. Learn more about this program at www.veteranaid. org.

Arizona Long-Term Care System (ALTCS). This is an Arizona Medicaid program under the Arizona Health Care Cost Containment System (AHCCCS). ALTCS pays for long-term care costs for those individuals and families who qualify, not only in nursing homes but also in assisted living homes and centers with which it is contracted. ALTCS also covers costs of some services in the senior's own home. To apply for ALTCS or to find more information, go to www. azahcccs.gov.

State and Private Resources

(Links to all websites listed below can be found at
www.careconnectionradionetwork.com)

Pima Council on Aging (PCOA) is a nonprofit advocacy organization that offers support to seniors. It has a variety of materials and educational programs available, as well as extensive resources to aid seniors in many situations. Learn more about how PCOA can serve you at www.pcoa.org.

Adult Protective Services (APS) is a division of the Arizona Department of Economic Security. This is the agency to contact should you encounter abuse, neglect, or exploitation of a vulnerable or elderly adult. Many times, an elderly adult will live alone and be unable to adequately care for himself, in which case APS can come in and help him negotiate a more appropriate living situation. It also can provide legal support and advice concerning powers of attorney, wills, trusts, and other fiduciary services. You can learn more about APS at www.azdes.gov/ aaa/programs/aps. To report any suspicion of abuse or neglect, call 1-877-SOS-ADULT (1-877-767-2385).

Department of Health Services (DHS). Division of Licensing Services/Assisted Living is the government department that licenses all assisted living facilities. DHS sends out surveyors to do annual inspections and follow up on complaints submitted by individuals or anonymously. Their website is www. azdhs.gov/als.

Ombudsman program is a division of the Arizona State Legislature. The ombudsman serves as an advocate for the elderly. If there is a situation that you cannot resolve with a loved one, a care center, or any aspect of your loved one's care journey, you can contact the long-term care ombudsman's office for help in finding solutions. The office can be contacted through www.azdes.gov and www.azdhs.gov.

Referral and placement agencies can help you choose an assisted living facility. There are two types—national and locally owned. Large national companies usually subcontract with agents or offer franchises in your area. These companies usually have a large Internet presence and do most of their business on the web. The other group is made up of smaller individually owned agencies that network with hospitals and rehab centers in addition to marketing their services in other ways. Both types of agents collect information from clients seeking care and generally do not charge the client a fee. They contract with homes and centers that agree to pay a fee for any resident placed in the facility. Locally owned and operated agencies tend to be more familiar with the homes and centers. Beware of agencies that cast the care industry in a bad light and promote fear and mistrust. Many of these will refer you to the home that pays the highest fee, regardless of quality of care.

3

Finding a Home: The Process

Finding an assisted living situation for your family member should be done carefully to reduce stress on everyone involved. A step-by-step process will help you to be objective and thorough in making your decision. It is important to involve your loved one in the process whenever you can. When this isn't possible, be sure to get input from everyone involved who knows your loved one well and understands his or her preferences. What follows is an outline of a process you might follow, but you can add and change steps as your situation warrants:

Quality of life. What is most important to Dad, you, and all those involved in this process? Decide what is most important to his quality of life. Do this before you begin looking, so that you won't lose sight of these considerations during the process. You may be dazzled by a number of extras that really don't contribute to what are the most important needs you've defined.

Prioritizing factors most important. You will need to consider various factors when choosing an appropriate facility. Price, location, room size, private vs. shared bath, private vs. semiprivate room, and services included in the rate are all things to think about. Before you start your search, prioritize which of these are most important to your situation. Also consider the unique needs of your loved one, and be sure the facility can accommodate those.

Conducting a search. Look on the DHS website and find homes in your zip code or area of preference (www.azdhs.gov/als). Call and visit as many facilities as you can to get a feel for what is available. If you wish to use the services of a referral agent, do so. As you conduct your search, you can go to the following website and find how each home and center has fared during its annual state survey: www.azdhs.gov/als/hcb/index.htm. Click on "Facility Search Including Inspection Reports." You will need the name or address of the specific facility in which you are interested.

Understanding the survey. All state-licensed facilities must pass an initial survey or inspection before obtaining a license. After that, they are inspected either annually or every two years. The home is issued a new license once the application is submitted and fees are paid, and then the state surveyor is free to come and inspect any time during the next year. If the home is found deficiency-free, the inspection is waived for the following year.

As with all systems, this is designed to bring accountability to the service providers and verify that they are operating within the intent of the law. Surveys are like tax audits. Many of us would not do well on a tax audit if we had no warning. We may not keep our accounts completely up-to-date throughout the year, but if we are responsible, we manage to catch up by April 15. If we are honest all year and keep reasonable notes, tax time is not such a challenge. Surveys are much like this. Keep in mind that surveyors are human and vary in their personalities. Some are more forgiving than others. Some give suggestions, where others might issue a deficiency. They operate within a set of legal boundaries, but a fairly wide area is open to subjective interpretation.

Kinds of deficiencies. The DHS website will tell you which homes have deficiencies and which do not, as well as which homes have had penalties or civil violations. It is very difficult to complete a survey with no deficiencies, so you are right to be impressed when a home manages that. That said, however, you need to know that just as it's possible to cheat on your taxes, there are ways to be deficiency-free at inspection time and substandard the rest of the year. Just because the home has no deficiencies doesn't mean things are in order all the time. Don't let survey results be your only guide to the quality of the home.

When you're touring, look for signs that all is in order. Pay close attention to how the residents of the facility look and act. You can get additional information from appendix 1 of this book, which has a list of things to check that will indicate whether the home functions at that standard year-round. Understand that some homes are administratively excellent but don't provide the warm and caring environment that will maximize the residents' quality of life. Look for the right balance of formal and informal qualities.

If you visit a home and feel good about it but find that it has deficiencies, consider what those deficiencies are and how they were reconciled. Discuss the issues with administrators and staff. If they give you satisfactory answers, you can feel reassured. Often, a mark or a citation results in a much stronger home. Deficiencies can be seen as educational tools for the home. With improvements in the quality of administrators and staff, problems can be resolved, and the home environment improved.

Overall management. The operations of a facility are affected as much by behind-the-scenes levels of management as by day-to-day operations. Consider these in your selection.

Owner Involvement

It is important to understand the role of the home's owner. There is a difference between the mom-and-pop operation, where the owner is there 24/7 and does a lot of the work, and the large corporation, where the owner lives elsewhere and oversees from a distance. Although neither scenario is ideal, either scenario can work, but you must adjust your expectations accordingly. Generally, homes where owners are involved are stronger overall. The buck stops with the owner. If he or she is available, approachable, and visible, this is a huge plus. No one loves your kids like you do, no one cares for your money like you do, and no one will care for a business like the owner. The owner may not pull shifts or provide actual care, but you should consider it a red flag if he or she is not engaged in any way.

Financial Viability

Don't hesitate to ask questions related to the business aspect of the facility. It may be the greatest provider in town, but if it goes bankrupt the week you move your loved one in, it's a bad situation. While you may not be able to look at account statements, feel free to ask questions such as:

- Have you ever missed a payroll?

- Do you have liability insurance?

- What is your staffing ratio?

- What type of staffing does the ratio include?

- Does the home adhere to the current code requirements?

Later in this chapter, we will discuss costs involved in running a home and define reasonable expectations.

Referral Agents

Referral agents are individuals who help you find an assisted living home or center. Their services are free to you because the facility where they place your loved one pays them a fee. Referral agents' qualifications vary greatly, as does their ability to find just the right facility for your mom. Good ones are in and out of facilities all the time. They tend to know what various places offer and what types of residents live there. Referral agents are in business to find a home for your loved one. Your understanding of the agent's role will empower you and enable you to make the best use of her time and talent. Take time to interview several agents and learn their qualifications and level of experience. Then choose the one who can best meet your needs.

At present, the referral agent system in Arizona is lightly regulated, though no accredited certification exists. Assisted living facilities, however, need to follow regulations that are related to referral agents. They are as follows:

- A facility must disclose to the residents and their representatives if it pays a fee to an agent.

- Assisted living licensed managers cannot take a fee for bringing a resident into the home they manage.

- The state prohibits any additional fee from being passed on to the resident if a family chooses to use a referral agent.

The agent does not charge the family but instead charges the facility for each placement. Some referral agents tour with the family and provide genuine guidance and support. Others merely hand out a list of phone numbers, and the family tours alone. A few might assist with discharge from the hospital, transportation to the facility, and other aspects of the transition.

Hospitals and rehabilitation centers generally will not directly refer a patient to an individual facility in order to avoid potential future liability. Referral agents are therefore the first to receive a name of someone looking for placement. Homes not listed with the referral agent you choose will not be shown.

Understanding the Costs Involved

Costs are a critical subject to discuss. You might spend between $3,500 and $9,000 a month for one bedroom (sometimes a shared bedroom) in a house or other facility, so the fees can seem rather steep. It is important to understand what that fee has to pay for.

Lois and Frank's Story

The strain was beginning to show on the faces of the five adult children caring for their aging parents. Frank and Lois had been married for almost 15 years. He was 97 years old and had lost his wife of 52 years 20 years earlier. He had two sons. Lois was 88. She had been married for 20 years before her husband was killed in a car accident. Lois had a son and two daughters.

Frank and Lois had been very good for each other. He suffered from a very slowly progressing Parkinson's disease that was well controlled with medication. Lois was in very good health, except for a slight cholesterol problem that she managed with a good diet and a few pills. It was clear the couple loved each other dearly.

Frank's greatest desire was to be allowed to age and die in his home of many years. He had watched his first wife suffer in a nursing home as cancer slowly robbed her of life before finally releasing her from this world. He had watched helplessly and felt completely powerless to change anything, as he was tossed to and fro in the wild sea of the medical system.

Life was ideal until the accident. As Frank's Parkinson's gradually became worse, Lois had taken on more of the role of caregiver. One day, Frank fell. Fortunately, nothing was broken, but he was in a great deal of pain and unable to get out of bed. Lois's blood pressure had been borderline high and recently had crept up to dangerous levels—the stress of caring for Frank and seeing his pain and suffering became too much for her, and Lois suffered a stroke. After she spent two weeks in the hospital and an-other two weeks in rehab, she was ready to come home.

The family had taken turns caring for Frank while they researched their options. Both parents were enrolled in hospice, so hospice nurses and shower aides came to their home to offer support. But that didn't begin to touch the 24/7 need for assistance with toileting, meals, house-keeping, and other care. It was a considerable challenge as well to navigate around their tiny house using wheelchairs and walkers.

Tensions were high, and tempers were short. The cost of round-the-clock care in their home was nearly $30,000 a month, and though all five kids wanted to do what was ab-solutely best for their parents, they couldn't afford to keep that up for more than a couple of months without throwing everyone into bankruptcy.

⟶ KEY POINT ⟵

A private room in assisted living is a better value than in-home care because care costs are shared among multiple residents.

Frank's and Lois's children were learning a very expensive lesson about the costs of in-home health care. To put it in perspective, paying for 24-hour care in your own home will cost a minimum of $14,500 a month. That's $20 an hour, times 24 hours a day, times 365 days a year, divided by 12 months—and it's hard to find someone for $20 an hour. In addition to that, you're paying the mortgage or rent, utilities, taxes, groceries, and so on. Then you still have to manage the caregivers. What do you do when they call in sick? What about the issues of liability if a caregiver is injured while caring for your loved one, or the complications of complying with proper IRS reporting rules?

Another option is to hire an agency to provide caregivers (who often have minimal training), but then the price will be $30 to $40 an hour, or $22,000 or more a month, in addition to the basic living expenses. Suddenly, $5,000 to $7,500 a month for housing, food, activities, and care looks more reasonable. Furthermore, there are many homes where your loved one will receive much better care than you may find from an agency, and the homes almost always are wheelchair-accessible. And don't forget the benefit of socialization with other people that assisted living offers.

A private room for $5,000 is very reasonable, as the costs are considerable on the provider's side. Staffing accounts for at least 50 percent of what a home brings in. The facility must pay for mortgage, utilities, liability insurance, taxes, the endless maintenance and upgrades necessary to maintain a healthy environment, and empty rooms and a referral fee to get them filled, not to mention groceries and other supplies for the residents. Five thousand dollars each for 10 residents is just about the minimum required to provide the quality care that most of us want for our loved ones.

As you shop for a home, cheaper rooms can be very appealing, and these facilities might provide outstanding care, but you must find out where they are cutting corners. Is the staff paid adequately? Is there a high staff turnover? What is the ratio of staff to residents? Is the staff that works during the night allowed to sleep? (If your loved one is up several times at night, this could be an issue.) What is the menu like? Is the facility maintained adequately? Is the owner working around the clock and ready to burn out? What types of activities and entertainment are offered? Often, a home can provide excellent care on a shoestring because the owner or manager is very thrifty and conscientious. Conversely, a home can be overpriced and still cut the same corners.

⟶ Key Point ⟵

When cost is an issue, you can provide services that the home cannot afford to offer, such as bringing in extra goodies, taking your loved one out, or sending in a sitter to play games or otherwise provide extra attention.

Be observant, investigate, and know what you're paying for. Know where you can fill in on your loved one's behalf to enhance his or her well-being, such as supplementing the menu with homemade goodies you know Grandma loves or bringing a stash of Dr.

Pepper for Dad. You might send a sitter in to play favorite games or read to Uncle Joe, or take Aunt Sally on a weekly outing to the beauty salon or movies. There are many ways to enhance your loved one's situation over what the facility provides. The key is clarifying your expectations, as will be discussed in the next chapter.

Important Consideration for This Season of Life

This book would not be complete without a segment on the significance of the final few years of life. As an individual approaches the end, every day becomes a huge percentage of the rest of her life. When considering what is best for your loved one, please see that these final days, months, and years are as comfortable as humanly possible. This is not the time to save money. If someone you love is in an unsatisfactory situation, don't let him stay there just to use up the cost of the 30 days' notice or for other financial reasons. No amount of money is worth your loved one's suffering during the final days of life. If you feel the end is near, a few hundred dollars a month of difference between a very high-quality place and a budget place that is inadequately staffed will not amount to much in exchange for a pleasant journey to the finish line.

When the Money Runs Out

Money will be a problem for many people facing long-term care. They may have outlived their savings or for whatever reason, it simply isn't there. When the money is gone, ALTCS, funded by Medicaid and the state, may be a viable option. Your loved one may qualify for this program when she is out of or close to being out of money. Once on ALTCS, any income, Social Security, or pension payments are turned over to the state, as are all assets. The state then takes over payment for all long-term care services. The person then gets a small monthly stipend for personal items.

Private pay almost always will secure a better environment. When government money is involved, bureaucracy increases. ALTCS limits your options dramatically, because many homes choose not to accept ALTCS funds in order to avoid the added complexity and inconvenience, lower revenues, added liability insurance requirements, and increased oversight that come with this program. Increased scrutiny doesn't necessarily mean that the quality will be better. It means that more time will be devoted to "proving" that standards are being met, which is not the same thing as providing quality care.

ALTCS pays flat rates for residents who qualify at three different levels of care. The monthly rate varies, but it is somewhere around $3,500 a month. ALTCS will pay only for a semi-private or shared room.

Some assisted living homes will let families pay privately for the difference in cost between a shared and private room. Homes providing more than two ALTCS beds are hard-pressed to staff adequately and provide the standard of care most of us would want.

If you find yourself needing this type of financial assistance, understand that an ALTCS placement may mean you will need to adjust your expectations. Your family can help make up for a lot in these situations. If the home can meet the resident's basic needs of food, housing, supervision, cleanliness, and medication management, the family can meet the need for social interaction, activity, and entertainment. The family also might pay for a companion to come in for the resident and take him out if he is able, play games, read books, or just provide company.

➤ KEY POINT ➤

Not all assisted living providers accept ALTCS. You may want to consider this before opting for it.

Long-Term Care Insurance

Long-term care insurance is great if you have it. The facility may need to meet certain requirements, depending on the policy. Some policies require that the home be licensed for 10 beds, or have an RN on staff or possibly on call. Generally, there's an assessment by a nurse, the home completes some paper-work, and then their invoice is sent to the insurance company monthly. Keep in mind that insurance companies pay after the service is rendered, while facilities charge in advance. Therefore, you should be prepared to pay up front and receive the reimbursement later. This type of insurance can take a huge weight off the family by greatly reducing, if not eliminating, the overwhelming costs associated with long-term care. You can get a list of companies that offer this type of insurance by visiting our website at www.integratedglobal.coach.

Caring for Mom at Home

People often opt for taking care of a family member at home. This can be a great option. We have seen some of our own residents go through rehabilitation from an accident or injury and return home to live very happily with a family who can meet their needs. Maybe there are grandkids or stay-at-home spouses available so that Grandpa isn't home alone and has the company and supervision he needs to be happy and content.

Be aware, however, that coming home also may lead to disaster. When families try to care for their aging loved ones at home, the loved ones often are neglected more than would be tolerated in even the worst of care facilities. It's not that the families don't care, but the reality is that we live in a busy society, where both husband and wife work outside the home or are involved in activities that require them to be out of the house.

Maybe you know someone who says, "Oh, I take care of my mom at home. She can't walk, but I just tell her to stay in her chair until I get home [maybe 8 hours later], and she does fine." This is *not* fine. An assisted living homeowner would go to jail if he took this attitude, and Adult Protective Services could be called in if the family does this. Be reasonable if you want to care for your parent at home. Know what you can and cannot do. Know what he or she needs, and be sure you can provide it.

Another consideration when caring for family at home is the health of the caregiver. One spouse can completely ruin his or her own health while caring for the other. A study conducted through Ohio State University and the University of North Carolina produced strong evidence that the continuing stress of providing in-home care can cause severe, long-term damage to the immune system of the caregiver. For more information—and some very interesting reading—go to www.researchnews.osu.edu/search.htm and enter "caregiver fatigue" in the search box.

➤ KEY POINT ➤

When choosing in-home care services, find agencies that have safeguards in place, such as training, fingerprint screening, and background checks for their caregivers.

Many agencies will send a caregiver into your home to help out. If what you need is supervision or assistance for a few hours a day, this can be an excellent solution. The cost will be comparable to 24-hour care in a facility, and you can still have Mom close by. Some long-term care insurance policies will cover this type of service.

Be aware that in Arizona, agencies that provide home caregivers are unregulated. You need to be diligent and observant. Find agencies that have safeguards in place, such as training, fingerprint screening, and background checks for their caregivers.

In the next chapter, we will discuss how to function within the assisted living system and about the many adjustments you and your loved one will encounter.

— 4 —

Functioning in the System

Entering the System

The process of moving a loved one into an assisted living facility varies widely from family to family and from situation to situation. Only the family, a responsible party, or an intimate friend can decide the best way to help an individual make that transition. Moving into a long-term care setting can be a breath of fresh air if one is coming from an institutional setting or anywhere that basic needs were not met. It also can entail an enormous sense of loss if the person moves from a home where he or she has lived for many years. Fortunately, there are many good options out there. The transition does not have to mean life is over.

⟍ KEY POINT ⟍

Moving into long-term care can entail an enormous sense of loss of freedom, privacy, independence, space, and property. It is important for all involved to be sympathetic toward the feelings and fears of the person who is moving.

Regardless of your individual situation, it's very important for all involved to be sympathetic toward the feelings and fears of the person who is moving into long-term care. Feelings of loss of freedom, privacy, independence, space, and property can be huge. These are very real fears when a vulnerable adult places herself in the care of complete strangers, many of whom look very different from the people to whom she is accustomed.

Whatever can be done to alleviate those fears should be done. We always suggest that the manager or owner of the facility meet the prospective resident so that the family has a face to associate with the new home. This can set Mom at ease and alleviate many fears. Also, if possible, bring the resident into the home for lunch or an activity in order to see who the new housemates and caregivers will be. Not only will this set Mom at ease if she likes what she sees, but it also can prevent a poor placement or poor fit into a community that is ultimately not going to work. As homeowners, we welcome this almost as much as the good fit, because of the problems that occur when a resident moves in who is not appropriate for our setting.

Every home and community has its own personality. We see this among staff and residents in the homes that we own. One place is a sanctuary for one person, while for another it can be completely intolerable. Encourage the prospective resident to be as involved as possible in the transition.

Know Your Family Member

We find there basically are three types of residents. You will know which category your loved one fits into, and thinking about that ahead of time will help you in your relationship with the facility and will contribute to your loved one's happiness. Regardless of the category in which they fall, all human beings deserve to be treated with dignity and respect. There is never a valid excuse for neglect, abuse, or mistreatment in any care setting. The following are the three general types of assisted living residents:

Never happy, no matter what. You try and try to make the person happy, but he will have none of it! The bed is always too hard or too saggy; the chair is all wrong; and the food is just ... well ... "*How do you expect me to eat this slop?*" The house is either too hot or too cold. The caregiver has no common sense, and neither does the person's own son or daughter. Nobody can ever get anything right. Complaining almost seems to be the only thing that makes him happy. This category includes the confused and the truly paranoid, as well as the alert and oriented who are just plain cranky or difficult.

What you must know about this person in the long-term care system is that he is very likely a target for abuse or neglect. If this is your loved one, it is very important that you communicate frequently with the facility staff and make sure that you all understand the nature of the resident. If the person is a habitual complainer, let the staff know you understand that, but at the same time, be alert to signs of abuse or neglect. Caregivers are human and may easily overlook the person who is likely to ruin their day. That person, however, is a vulnerable adult and deserves to be cared for and looked after. Find a few things (personal or food items, activities, music) that you know your loved one truly appreciates and make every effort to supply them.

Completely content no matter what. This person is very easy to love. No one can do wrong. She is completely understanding and tolerant of uncomfortable beds, poor chairs, and lousy food. She understands that nobody's perfect and extends grace to the clumsy caregiver, forgetful son or daughter, or obnoxious fellow resident. (This type of person is probably married to the "never happy, no matter what" person, by the way.) She smiles and says thank you and rarely is a trouble. This is the person every care home wants to take care of. This person also can be overlooked and neglected, however, simply because she is not a squeaky wheel. If this is your loved one, encourage her to communicate her wants and needs. You also should feel free to tell the staff about needs that Mom feels comfortable sharing with you but not with them.

Happy as long as a few key needs are met. This is the category into which most of us fit. For the most part, if a few key expectations are met, we can live contentedly and get along. For most of us, though, without certain things, life can really stink. Maybe it's that fresh-ground cup of coffee right when you wake up or the afternoon martini you've been enjoying for the past 60 years. We have developed a brief quality-of-life questionnaire (appendix 2) that helps to identify these core needs. If the home you're considering doesn't have something like this in place, you might want to complete the form so that your expectations are clear and in writing. In the beginning, follow up frequently to make sure the routines that are in place take these things into account.

Communication and Developing a Team

Caring for Mom, Once Settled

A mistake many people make is thinking that once you have secured a location for your loved one, you can now become disengaged. Not so! It is very important to accompany your loved one through the system. Just as no one will love your children the way you do, and no one will care about your money the way you do, no one will love your mom and dad the way you do. That doesn't mean that caregivers won't take care of Mom and Dad as well as you would; it just means that even in the best of facilities, people are fallible, and important things can get overlooked. The more people there are who focus on Mom, the better off she will be. Any good facility will welcome your insights, suggestions, and overall input. Also, your presence will most likely result in improved staff performance overall.

Building a Relationship with the Caregiving Team

The best way to ensure quality care is to build a relationship with the caregiving team. Every business and social network has both its angels and its demons. Please, for your family member's sake, be an angel in the system in which you find yourself. This will make a huge difference in the way people respond to you and Mom.

⟶ KEY POINT ⟶

Be an angel in the system in which you find yourself. This will make a huge difference in the way people will respond to you and your family member.

A good relationship with the facility depends primarily on three things: honest communication, kind communication, and respectful communication. Careful communication will do more than any team of lawyers and doctors to promote the comfort and care of your family member. Respect the team as a group of people who generally are underpaid for the value they offer. They do what they do mostly because they genuinely care about their residents and reap great nonmonetary rewards for their work. But there are exceptions to every rule. If problems arise, waste no time in addressing them calmly, and chances are they will never reach crisis level.

The Communication Triangle

We designed this communication triangle as a way to see how communication needs flow and where the accountability lines are, in order to provide the highest quality of life possible to our residents — we are all in this business for that one reason. It's imperative that the balance always be in place. At times, the staff may play the family against the owner, or the family may pit the resident against the staff, or there might be many other dysfunctional scenarios. But the only way to ensure that the resident's quality of life will be maintained is if the lines of communication are functioning well.

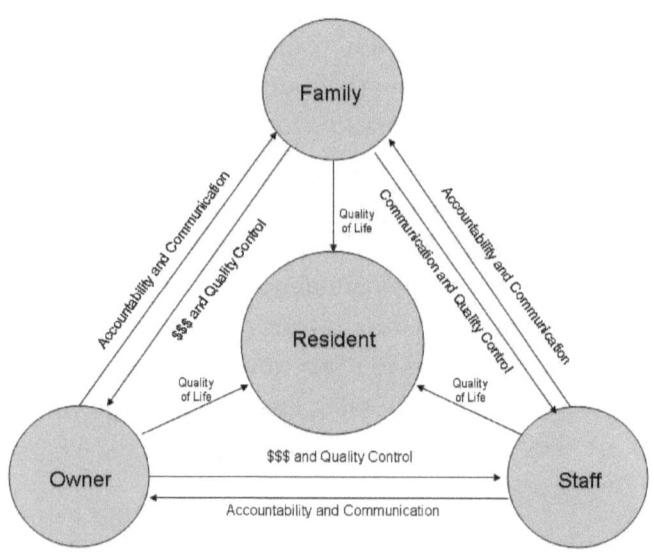

You may want to use the triangle as a tool to initiate communication with the manager or owner of the facility. Find out what she does to keep the lines open and what accountability structures are in place. If you have a problem with a caregiver or another resident, address it with the manager. If that doesn't bring about the results you need, what does the facility want you to do next?

In our homes, we make ourselves available to ensure that such problems are corrected. It works very well. The manager doesn't always have the resources or the authority to make the corrections, so the team should include an active owner or an administrator who carries the authority to solve problems.

Setting Realistic Expectations

Setting realistic expectations begins with understanding and providing what your loved one needs and wants. For instance, you may eat a very healthy diet, while Mom might love white bread and gravy. It's important to recognize that this is all about Mom's quality of life and meeting her needs and desires. Also, keep in mind that personalized care in assisted living must be a balance of the best interests of all the residents. To achieve this goal, you must openly communicate your expectations to determine if the home can accommodate them. There are, however, two areas that tend to require a little more careful attention: food and activities.

Food is always a hot topic in assisted living. A facility must consider not only the cost of food but also its residents' health needs and their preferences. Just because you want your loved one to eat healthy doesn't mean he will, even if offered healthy choices. This doesn't mean that only unhealthy foods should be offered, either. The facility needs to offer a balance between health needs and food preferences. Review the menus, and if you don't feel there's a balance, talk to the manager.

Consider this true story: *Mary* (not her real name) *lived at a large assisted living center that offered freshly baked cookies every day. She really looked forward to the afternoons when the cookies came out of the oven, and she could enjoy a warm one with milk. Mary had no cognitive impairment, so she was able to make decisions regarding her care. After a few months at the center, she had put on a few pounds, probably from eating those delicious cookies, which upset her health-conscious daughter. One day, the daughter stormed in to the director's office and demanded that the director prohibit Mary from eating the cookies, or the daughter would report the center to the Department of Health Services! The director pointed out that even though the daughter had power of attorney, she couldn't make decisions for her mom until her mom was declared incompetent. The director also pointed out how much Mary loved the cookies and what joy it brought her to eat them. The daughter left the office indignantly. The next day, the director received a call from the Department of Health Services, saying the facility had been reported for "having freshly baked cookies" every day, which was causing their residents to gain weight. The director explained what had happened with the woman's daughter the previous day. The surveyor laughed and said he wouldn't come out to investigate and would list the complaint as unsubstantiated. The moral of the story is that we all have freedom of choice, unhealthy or not.*

Assisted living state regulations require that activities be provided and an activity calendar be posted. You may find there is a direct correlation between the monthly cost and the type of activities offered. For example, an expensive facility might have a harpist once a month, whereas a less costly facility might do karaoke instead. Again, this is about balance between residents' preferences and cost. Keep in mind that Mom probably doesn't listen to a harpist once a month at home or do karaoke either, so look for a place that accommodates the type of activities that Mom likes, rather than what sounds fun to you. Also, consider the type of person that Mom is and what makes her feel well cared for. If she's social, then make sure she's out of her room and engaged with someone for most of the day. But if she's an introvert, you would want to provide things to do in her room and then encourage her to be out for brief periods.

How Things Work

Certain rules and regulations govern assisted living facilities. What follows are a few things you should know about what the law requires. You can learn more about the DHS regulations through its website or by visiting assistedlivingmarketplace.org and linking to AZ DHS.

Tuberculosis, Pneumonia, and Flu

Before you move your loved one into an assisted living facility, you will need to provide proof that she is free from tuberculosis. This can be determined by a chest X-ray or a skin test that has been done within the last 6 months. The form, signed by the doctor or nurse, must state that the person is free from TB. It cannot merely say *no active disease* or *normal* or something of that nature. Be sure to notify your doctor or hospital staff that you need this before moving your relative.

The facility is required by law to make flu and pneumococcal vaccines available to its residents annually. Your loved one can forgo these vaccinations; you just need to notify the facility in writing.

The Service Plan

Within 14 days of move-in, according to Arizona law, assisted living facilities must prepare a service plan, also called a care plan, outlining the nature of the care the facility will provide. The manager, a registered nurse, or a nurse practitioner will prepare the plan. In the case of a directed-care resident or when the caregivers will be giving medications, a nurse must prepare the plan. There is generally an additional charge to you for this service, and you should be asked to participate in and sign the care plan.

The plan defines exactly what services the home will provide to assist with medication and activities of daily living. The law states that the plan must be updated whenever there are significant changes, such as those that may occur after hospitalization or severe illness. It also must be updated every 3, 6, or 12 months, depending on level of care. There usually is a charge each time the plan is updated, because the nurse has to come to the home and do an assessment.

Under Lock and Key

Assisted living regulations were designed to protect people, including those with dementia who may have poor judgment. As a result, any product (including toothpaste, lotions, and mouthwash) that has a warning label or reads "Keep out of the reach of children" must be kept in a locked receptacle. This can seem very restrictive for seniors who have no cognitive impairment. You can talk to the owner about putting a cabinet or box with a lock in Mom's room or putting a lock on the door. Then, anything in her room is considered secure when the door is locked. State regulations also require that the caregivers have a key.

The Chain of Command

In an assisted living situation, the staff must abide by *doctor's orders*. These are maintained on a form stating which medications and treatments the resident may and must receive, dosages, times, and any special instructions. Some meds are ordered regularly, such as blood pressure medicine; others are PRN (as needed), such as acetaminophen for a headache. The facility is obligated to follow doctor's orders.

Often, family members will want to make changes or withhold a medication. They may disagree with the physician. Even if you hold medical power of attorney, you may not instruct the caregiver or staff to violate doctor's orders. If you wish to make a change, discuss it with the doctor, who then can issue new orders. The staff cannot give any medication that is not listed on the orders, and they must give those that are ordered. Because of potential drug interactions, the use of alcohol must be approved by doctor's order as well.

Advance Directives

DNR: The Do-Not-Resuscitate Order

When you place your loved one in long-term care, you will be asked about his end-of-life wishes and whether he wants to receive CPR or other life-support measures, should his heart or breathing stop.

One option is *Full Code*, meaning that if his heart stops, all measures will be taken to revive him. Another option is *Do Not Resuscitate (DNR)*, meaning that if the heart and/or breathing stops, CPR or other life-support methods will not be used, and nature will take its course. You can learn more about how this affects your loved one by talking to his or her doctor.

If your loved one does not want to be resuscitated, then the home or her physician will ask you to complete an orange DNR form. This form tells paramedics your loved one's wishes. *It is only valid for paramedics.* If your loved one chooses the DNR option, she also should have an advanced directive (discussed below). Of course, this doesn't mean that if a person is choking on a hot dog, the staff will stand by and let him die or that they won't call the paramedics if it looks like she's having a stroke. It merely means that if the staff or paramedics see that a person's heart or breathing has stopped, they will not perform CPR or otherwise try to bring the person back.

The Living Will and Related Issues

It is extremely important to find out your loved one's end-of-life wishes while she still can tell you what they are. This is especially important if your loved one does not want advanced life-support measures. Careconnectionradionetwork.com contains links to many valuable resources that can help you do this. Medical and financial powers of attorney should be obtained in the event that your loved one reaches a point at which she is unable to make decisions for herself. Individuals may assign someone power of attorney, but the *power to make decisions for them exists only if the individuals are not able to make decisions for themselves.*

The living will, or advance directive, is a document that outlines what your loved one's end-of-life and resuscitation wishes are. You can request a Life Care Planning Packet from the Arizona Attorney General's website to learn more. Another valuable resource that all authorities in Arizona respect is *The Five Wishes*. This document walks you through each major decision regarding care and issues related to end of life. Your loved one—in fact, every adult—should have a copy and should keep it updated. Be sure your loved one signs it and has it witnessed; your loved one also may choose to have this form notarized, so there is no question of its validity. (Some states require that this form be notarized.) *The Five Wishes* can be purchased at www.agingwithdignity.org, or you can obtain a free copy through our website, www.integratedglobal.coach. Whether you choose *Five Wishes* or a different advance directive, make sure that your loved one's home has a copy of the document.

Expectations and Quality of Life

What Is Reasonable?

It is important to identify core points that are necessary to your loved one's happiness before you select a home. Otherwise, you might be swayed into choosing a situation that ultimately will not suit him or her. It is important to communicate these points at the outset to the facility.

No facility can be everything to everyone, but any home can cater to a few important requests for each resident, if it makes those requests a priority. For example, maybe hot coffee at 5:00 AM is critical to Dad's having a good day, but bingo on Thursday is not at all to his taste. Perhaps Uncle Joe craves peanut butter and jelly with an ice-cold Coke at 2:00 AM, but he really doesn't like Sunday worship. Or Mom might say that Sunday worship is the only thing that keeps her going from week to week, but she hates coffee and only gets hungry at mealtimes. Identify what is important to your loved one, and tell the staff about these things. It is not unreasonable to expect the home to accommodate you.

What to Expect from a Large Center vs. a Home

Larger centers may not be able to give Mom as much personal attention as a smaller center would, but it can happen, and larger facilities can offer many things smaller homes cannot. You will have a bigger job of communicating with caregivers in a center, because it's a larger staff and more people will be directly caring for your mom. You may need to take on the role of quality-of-life manager and see to it that friends and family visit to help Dad feel secure and cared for.

Larger centers can offer a greater array of activities, such as transportation to shopping centers and other places, regular recreation, and restaurant-style dining. These points may impress you, but if they're not important to your loved one, then don't make them factors for choosing the right place to meet your loved one's needs.

Certain services should be offered by any assisted living facility. You should expect any facility to do the following:

- Accurately manage medications and treatments.

- Maintain a clean, odor-free environment.

- Serve balanced, nutritious, tasty meals and snacks.

- Respect the residents' dignity and rights, and treat them with kindness and common sense.

- Attempt to incorporate residents' personal interests and tastes into their activities and menus.

- Comply with all applicable DHS rules and regulations.

- Be receptive to communication from family and be willing to solve problems.

Assisted living facilities must provide three meals and a snack each day, activities, and care, which means assistance with activities of daily living. A large center might offer multiple food options at each meal, whereas a home would offer one option and possibly an alternative. Residents may not be able to request individualized meals, unless necessitated by a specialty diet ordered by a doctor. It's also not reasonable to expect the facility to provide meal replacement supplements or expensive foods on a routine basis.

Another difference between larger centers and homes is the number and variety of activities offered on a daily basis. A home will offer one or two activities a day versus a center, which might have five or six. Families often are more attracted to a higher number of activities, but residents usually only choose to participate in a maximum of one activity a day. It is crucial to keep Mom's needs and wants in mind, instead of your own.

Activities of daily living (ADLs) and assistance needed are defined in each resident's individualized service plan. The fees charged by a center or home are usually based on this plan. Caregivers cannot be expected to perform personal tasks for a resident beyond assistance with defined ADLs, according to that service plan. You can expect continuous one-on-one contact only if you're paying a private caregiver to come in for that.

Special services and items can be requested ahead of time, and the provider, the resident, and the family should agree on what is expected. Let's face it; personal attention is available at the right price. If you are willing to spend $15,000 a month or more, you can generally see to it that your loved one receives individual attention, personal services, and a varied menu at meals. If you feel your loved one needs a little extra TLC, you might consider hiring a companion for a few hours a week for an extra outing or one-on-one time. In addition, you may bring into the facility the special foods or drinks, such as soda, that your loved one wants to eat.

It is not reasonable to expect the facility to be perfect, but it is reasonable to expect consistent patterns of quality care. If the facility is not meeting your expectations, it is your responsibility to sit down with the manager to communicate and clarify expectations.

Abuse

When to Be Truly Concerned: Signs of Neglect and Abuse

Neglect and abuse can and do occur in assisted living facilities, and it's important to be able to recognize some signs, especially if your loved one is confused, difficult to manage, or unable to communicate. Some of the most likely targets of abuse are demanding, unkind, combative, or uncooperative residents.

It's often hard to identify incidents of actual abuse. One of the first signs of dementia is paranoia. Residents who are confused often become fearful and imagine things that are not true. It is especially difficult for those with dementia to distinguish the real from the merely perceived, as hallucinations are not uncommon in this illness. If you have concerns about abuse, discuss them with the manager or owner *immediately*. Here are some signs:

- Outright accusations. These need to be considered in context.

- Increasing fear of a particular person.

- Bruising or burns that look suspicious.

- Bedsores in otherwise healthy residents, except toward the end of life, as the body loses the ability to heal itself.

- Psychological changes, such as fear of abandonment or unusual attachment to a certain person.

Legal Responsibilities Regarding Abuse

Every care environment is governed by laws that obligate caregivers and staff to report any abuse they witness or suspect, even by visitors and family members. If an employee witnesses or suspects abuse, he has a legal obligation to report it to Adult Protective Services (APS). Failure to do so can result in fines and even arrest. APS then conducts an investigation and helps resolve problems that might have triggered the alleged abuse.

Families often have disagreements, and tempers can flair. It is always unacceptable to use abusive speech or actions toward a vulnerable adult. Withholding medication and treatments is considered negligence, and the family cannot fail to supply the facility with the means to carry out a doctor's orders.

Outside Services

Case Management

Sometimes it's difficult to navigate health care, especially if you're not in the same state as your loved one. A case manager may be able to help you and your loved one. Case managers are either specially trained social workers or nurses who focus on managing health care and other services. If you need help managing your loved one's doctors, treatments, and medications, choose an RN case manager. However, if you are comfortable managing the medical issues, then a social worker would be sufficient. Some case managers also can serve as guardians. In addition, a case manager can help connect you to other resources you may need, such as fiduciary help (someone to pay the bills and manage money), attorney services, or community resources.

RN Advocacy

Nurse advocacy is new to the health-care arena and expands on the services of a nurse case manager. An advocate helps ensure your loved one is receiving appropriate medical care. This type of professional also can battle with insurance companies to make sure appropriate medical services are provided. In addition, an advocate can be your eyes and ears while your family member is at the doctor or in the emergency room.

Medicare Home Health

Medicare provides for this type of skilled care in the assisted living facility or private home under qualifying circumstances. Skilled care means services provided by a licensed health-care professional, such as a registered nurse or a physical, occupational, or speech therapist. The home health benefit is free for covered services. Certified agencies can provide nursing, physical therapy, occupational therapy, speech therapy, and some assistance with bathing and other activities of daily living. Services are provided for a determined certification period and can continue as long as eligibility requirements are met. If your loved one is getting weaker or is not walking steadily, physical therapy could help. If your loved one is receiving new medications or treatments, a nurse can help make sure they're being delivered correctly. To get started, ask your loved one's doctor to send an order to a Medicare-certified home-care agency.

Medicare Hospice Benefit

Hospice is a great Medicare benefit that many people do not understand. It does not mean your loved one is going to die today or next week or even this year. And it doesn't mean your loved one won't continue to receive care. The general guideline for enrolling in hospice care is that there is a reasonable chance the person could pass away within the next 6 months. Generally speaking, enrolling in hospice says *I'm done fighting and trying to get better. I'm ready to let nature take its course. Please keep me comfortable.* Often, an individual will enroll in hospice services and, because of the increased attention the team approach provides, will improve and be discharged from hospice.

The hospice organization will do an evaluation at the request of the primary-care doctor and determine if the person is eligible. Weight loss, failure to thrive, and terminal diagnoses (such as chronic heart failure, stroke, multiple serious illnesses, and high risk of another heart attack) are some of the things that might make one eligible.

There are very good reasons for enrolling your loved one, especially as there are no co-pays or fees to use the Medicare hospice benefit. Hospice not only cares for the dying person but also offers grief counseling and coping support for the family and caregivers. This support continues for 13 months or more after your loved one passes. Hospice pays for certain medications, including those for pain and comfort care and those related to the admitting diagnosis, as well as incontinence supplies and added care assistance, such as a shower aide. Hospice provides an RN or LPN to visit the resident as often as necessary for his or her comfort and well-being. This added medical attention often leads to significant recovery, and many people are taken off hospice because they begin to improve and even thrive.

Some hospice agencies send out volunteers who will play games or just sit with your loved one to meet the need for social interaction. They also will assign a social worker to act as an advocate with the medical system and the management of the facility. Hospice can provide chaplains of all faiths for spiritual support.

Hospice is the only medical treatment that truly

uses a team approach to treat the patient and the family. Most important, however, is its focus on keeping the patient comfortable. Most of us want to be able to die with dignity and with minimal pain.

⇀ KEY POINT ⇀

On hospice, medications are available to alleviate pain and anxiety, allowing the patient to pass peacefully. Without hospice, it can be difficult to obtain palliative (comfort) medications in sufficient dosages to make the patient comfortable.

What Hospice Is Not

Hospice is not a death sentence. For instance, if Mom is in hospice for terminal cancer and she gets pneumonia, she certainly may opt to be treated for pneumonia. If Dad is on hospice for failure to thrive, and he falls and breaks a hip, he can choose to be taken immediately to the hospital to be treated, or he can remain where he is and receive comfort care. Once the decision is made to go to the hospital, your loved one might be discharged from hospice but can be readmitted later. Your loved ones will never be refused treatment because they are on hospice care, but certain treatments, such as physical therapy, can disqualify them from the program.

— 5 —

Ending Your Long-Term Care Experience

Your loved one might end his or her long-term care experience for any of several reasons, such as:

- Your loved one may improve and be able to return to living independently.

- You may be unhappy with the current facility or otherwise decide that a different facility will better meet your loved one's needs.

- Your loved one passes away, and services are no longer needed.

Knowing the following helpful points will make the transition less stressful:

Returning Home

What a joy when this happens! We have had people in our care go from hospice to thriving to moving back home. There are certain things to think about if this occurs. Know what your loved one's contract says regarding termination of the agreement. Most places require a 30-day written notice. It will make everyone's life easier if you do this, even if the contract does not require it. If your loved one moves out with less than 30 days' notice, the home may continue to charge for those days (this may be because it doesn't have enough time to advertise the room and get it filled—this is not unreasonable). Once Mom has given notice and moved out, she should be reimbursed any unused fees (as well as any security deposit) within 30 days.

Moving from One Facility to Another

Moving from rehab into an assisted living facility or from a lower level of care into a higher level is commonplace; it need not involve conflict. Moving because your loved one is unhappy, however, is a touchy situation that brings an added need for tact and etiquette. In either case, to ensure the smoothest transition possible, communicate very clearly to both the home Dad is leaving and the one into which he is moving. Sometimes people want to avoid conflict, so they leave without notice. This is not a good strategy. It is always better to use clear communication. If you are concerned about the reaction of the staff or feel they may try to talk you into staying, bring along an advocate who can stand up to them and who is not as emotionally involved. It can be a very sensitive issue, but you will better serve the needs of your loved one by doing things properly and being up front in your communications.

- Submit a letter of termination that includes your name, the date, the date of the move, and the reason for the move (if you want to include it). If you choose not to give 30 days' notice, be prepared to pay for the remaining days so that there are no difficulties down the line.

- Obtain copies of the care plan, signed doctor's orders, documentation of freedom from TB, all medications, lab reports as needed, and the original orange DNR (which should accompany the resident whenever he leaves the facility). You also may request copies of medication administration reports if you wish, but this is usually unnecessary. Be sure to keep copies of all the records you send to the new facility.

- Inform hospice or the nursing agencies caring for your loved one about the change. If equipment needs to be moved, such as a hospital bed or an oxygen concentrator, contact the company that owns it. They will usually want to move it themselves. They probably will issue new equipment and pick up the old one after the move.

- Upon arriving at the new facility, introduce Mom to the staff and to a few residents who may be out and about. If she's up to it, give her a short tour of her new home. Otherwise, show her to her room and let her lie down to rest, saving the tour for when she has more energy.

- To help her adjust, try highlighting things about her new home that you know she'll appreciate; for instance, an activity you know she'll enjoy or another resident with whom she'll be able to relate.

- Once Mom is settled, give copies of the above reports to the manager. Find out who is the best person to talk to about Mom's needs, likes, and dislikes. You can waste a lot of time telling the owners that Mom hates mayonnaise but really loves her 3:00 gin and tonic if they are not the ones who make her sandwich or plan happy hour.

When Your Loved One Passes Away

A little planning can make this time of loss for family and friends a lot more peaceful for everyone. Death is a reality, and plans that were made earlier, when you were all in your right minds, allow you to focus on your own grieving and the needs of family and friends.

Usually, the facility will charge for as many days as the resident's things are left in the room. It is a good idea to designate someone to move Dad's personal belongings out promptly. You will be very busy, and everyone will be grieving, but you might spend several hundred dollars unnecessarily by waiting a week to clear out the room.

The facility is obligated to refund any unused fees for the remainder of the month after the room is vacated. It has 30 days to refund your fees, petty cash, and deposit money.

— 6 —

Oh, No! I Didn't Plan!

You're Not Alone

Yes, we know you're out there—we see you every day. This section offers a step-by-step guide to handling critical issues, so that you can avoid major pitfalls. Still, we highly recommend reading the book cover to cover, which is why we made it short.

Step 1

If you need to place your loved one quickly, go to our website at www.integratedglobal.coach. There, you can fill out a brief questionnaire, and someone will contact you within 24 hours to discuss your needs and be your personal advisor.

Step 2

Obtain a TB skin test for your loved one. You will need this anywhere you go, and it takes at least 48 hours to read. You can get this at your primary healthcare provider's office or other clinic. If your loved one needs to move in less than 48 hours, you also can have him or her get a chest X-ray, which will produce immediate results. There are local companies that can even do the X-ray at your home.

Step 3

If possible, discuss with Mom and Dad what is most important to them. Some things that might lead you to a smaller home are personal care needs (toileting, transferring, fall risk), fully prepared meals, services like laundry and housekeeping, and medication management. If these are real needs, the smaller home is much better equipped to carry them out at a much higher standard, as it will almost always have a better ratio of staff to residents. A larger facility would cater better to a more independent individual who may need limited physical assistance but wants a larger social community and transportation to shopping and doctor visits. Because of the staff-to-resident ratio in larger facilities, residents will wait longer for assistance and are largely left on their own for socialization or participation in activities. If Mom or Dad requires more complex medical care, you may need to consider a skilled nursing facility.

Step 4

Determine how much the family is willing to spend. This will help tremendously in your search for a home. Remember that the costs (care, food, facility, licensing, insurance, etc.) are very real for the care institution, and you most likely will get only what you pay for and little else. If money is an issue, decide how the family can contribute to enhance what the facility is able to provide.

Step 5

If your time is short, you may benefit greatly from contacting a referral agent. The facility releasing your family member will most likely give you the name of someone who can help. You also can go to our website at www.integratedglobal.coach, and we will do our best to help you find a facility that meets your needs.

The Arizona Department of Health Services Assisted Living website lists the names and locations of homes, with their zip codes, and it also lists the most recent inspection reports online. You may want to check this site to make sure you aren't overlooking a good option nearby that may not be contracted with your referral agent.

A Final Word of Encouragement

Making the transition into a long-term care environment always involves a certain amount of anxiety, uncertainty, and stress. There will be a sense of loss of freedom and an end to life as you know it. We hope we have given you an idea of how the system works so that the transition will be a bit smoother.

You aren't alone—there are resources in the community for you. Our suggestion is that you and your family enter into this transition with an open heart. Welcome opportunities for growth, and look for new relationships that might even turn into lifelong friendships. Keep a positive attitude and find reasons to be grateful. Look for ways you can bring happiness to your loved one and to others in her new community. Only you can determine what you bring to the experience, and we hope that you will bring hope and optimism with you to your loved one's new home.

~ Appendix 1 ~

Evaluating Assisted Living Quality and Suitability

Evaluating assisted living is one of the trickiest things you will ever do for your loved one. Keep in mind that one of the best indicators of a good home is how you feel as you walk through the facility. Even if you cannot pinpoint why you feel good or bad about a place, take those feelings seriously. A bad feeling may be as simple as a personality conflict, but the high level of trust you must place in those caring for Mom or Dad will come a lot easier if your overall feeling is positive.

What follows are a few questions to ask the administration and staff of the facility. Questions to ask yourself as you tour are shown in italics. Note the details you feel are most important before you begin looking for a facility. And be sure to take notes—don't count on your memory in a time of stress.

ASK:

- What levels of care do you provide?

- Are there adequate safeguards in place for directed care?

- Are there secure outdoor areas for unattended residents?

- Is the staff equipped for my loved one's specific needs?

- What is the staffing ratio? Is that guaranteed?

- Is it all right if I drop in unannounced and roam around?

- How are wandering residents handled?

- What are the costs? What does that include? What are the added charges?

- Does the facility have nurse practitioners or doctors who visit? How often?

- What is their role in patient care? How are they paid?

- How are prescriptions handled?

- Is there a security deposit? Is it refundable? Is there a community fee?

- Do you provide transportation? If so, who drives and in what vehicle? Is transportation only on certain days? Is there an additional fee for transportation?

- Are electric wheelchairs allowed? What are the restrictions? Do they pose a hazard to mobility?

- What activities do you provide?

- Do people come in for special activities?

- Do you provide for spiritual needs?

- How are activities tailored to the needs and interests of the residents?

- Can residents choose between eating in their rooms or going to the dining room? Is there an extra charge if meals are taken to the room?

- How are food preferences and special diets handled? Is there an extra charge?

- What are the alcohol, smoking, and pet policies? (*Am I comfortable with these policies? How do I feel about pets on the premises?*)

OBSESRVE:

- Do the caregivers look like people with whom Mom will feel comfortable?

- Are they clean and dressed neatly?

- Are they alert and attentive?

- Do the residents look clean, cared for, and happy?

- At first glance, do I think Mom will get along with them?

- Does the food look appetizing? Are the meals healthful?

- What does the home smell like? Does it look and feel clean? Is the lighting adequate?

- Is the temperature comfortable? Do I think it will be comfortable for my family member?

- Is there a positive attitude in the home? Are residents out and about? [People might be napping at midmorning and midafternoon, so there would be less activity at those times. Observe the facility at different times of day.]

➤ Appendix 2 ➤

Quality-of-Life Care Plan

Name:_____

Likes to be called:_____

Favorite foods:_____

Food dislikes:_____

Activity preferences:_____

_____

Brief history of life and accomplishments:_____

_____

Quality-of-life factors *(Please list those things we can do to maximize the resident's quality of life)*:

_____

_____

_____

Quality-of-Life Care Plan (Sample)

Name: Cynthia Lou Adams

Likes to be called: Cindy Lou

Favorite foods: Mashed potatoes, tamales, and clam chowder

Food dislikes: Orange juice, grapefruit

Activity preferences: Loves to watch sitcoms on TV; hates sports programs; likes to play dominos and Scrabble; likes to do craft projects but needs assistance with small items.

Brief history of life and accomplishments: Married for 40 years, spouse deceased three years ago; two children, six grandchildren, and two great-grandchildren; was a field hospital nurse in Vietnam, then retired to raise her family. She was an active member of the Weaver's Guild until last year. When her children were young, she loved to enter her crafts and baked goods in competition at the Pima County Fair.

Quality-of-life factors *(Please list those things we can do to maximize the resident's quality of life)*:

Mom loves to be around animals and children, so if her dog could visit, she would really like it. She also loves to bake and would probably like to help in the kitchen.

⟶ Appendix 3 ⟶

Nonmedical Home Care Questionnaire

**(For use when contracting
with an in-home care agency)**

Deal-Breaker Questions

(if the answer is no, *don't use that agency!)*

Yes　No　　1.　Are background checks or
fingerprinting done on *every* caregiver?

Yes　No　　2.　If hands-on care is needed, is the
caregiver a certified nursing assistant
(CNA) or certified caregiver, or has
the caregiver had at least 24 hours of
training?

Yes　No　　3.　Do caregivers keep a communication
log or notes so I will be able to learn
what's going on with my loved one
when I'm not there?

Useful Information You Need to Know

4. How is this company different from other companies offering the same services?

5. What are the hourly rates? Sitter/companion:_____ Caregiver:_____

6. What's the minimum hours per day and week to use the service?_____

Yes   No   7.   Are rates higher for nights, weekends, or holidays?

Yes   No   8.   Is there a lower rate if the caregiver can sleep at night?

Yes   No   9.   Is a supervisor available, by phone, 24/7, if needed?

10. How do you monitor caregiver attendance/time?

— Appendix 4 —

Sample Emergency Information

Name:_____

Date of Birth:_____

Emergency Contact:_____

Cell Phone:_____

Alternate Contact:_____

Cell Phone:_____

Doctor:_____

Phone:_____

Allergies:_____

Hospital:_____

Health problems/diagnosis:_____

_____

_____

Pacemaker, internal defibrillator, implants:_____

_____

_____

Special religious needs:_____

_____

_____

_____

Medications, vitamins, supplements:_____

_____

_____

_____

Acknowledgments

We would like to acknowledge those who have made the writing of this book possible. First, we thank God for the incredible opportunity He has given us to work in this industry and to participate in the lives of so many people at such a profound time. We have been so blessed and enriched as a result. We also thank Him for the strength to make it through the rough times—and there have been many—and for the subsequent growth and maturity He brought about in our lives as a result. It has been through the development of our business that we have gained the education and knowledge to produce this book.

We would also like to thank our kids, Samuel, Jonathan, and Katie, for their incredible ability to hang in there and become amazing young adults and for the contributions of hard work, ideas, and moral support that they have given over the years. We could not have built this business without their help, patience, and understanding on so many occasions.

We must thank the Arizona Homestead residents, staff, and families who have educated us from the beginning. We started with very little knowledge of long-term care or of running a business, but we have learned along the way and have appreciated those who have been there and given us the opportunity to serve them as we learned, sometimes by trial and error.

Finally, we would like to say thank you to the Arizona Department of Health Services for its support of those caring for our seniors. We truly feel that in being there for our residents, the DHS is there for us and helps our success as we work as a team to provide the highest possible quality of life for those in our community.

About the Authors

Tammy Burns

It is an unusual woman with an unusual passion for people who would be willing to raise her children in a foreign land and then return home to build a business from zero for the sake of serving others. Tammy and her family spent seven years working for a non-profit agency, training leaders in Brazil and around the world, before returning to Tucson, where she has poured herself into learning what it takes to run a business and take care of vulnerable adults at the highest possible level. Since 2004, she and her family have established several lasting healthcare businesses in Tucson. After leaving the formal business arena in Arizona, and living part time overseas, Tammy has continued to pursue her passion for people through becoming a personal trainer and life coach. She offers these services through her new business, Integrated Global Coaching and Consulting.

Russell Burns

Over the years Russell's experience in the senior care industry, both for and not for profit, led him to become a leading voice for seniors in Arizona. He and his family worked to establish leading senior care organizations that are still raising the standard in senior care today. Today he and Tammy are active with Integrated Global Coaching and Consulting, where they continue to help people and organizations navigate their journeys.

Cindy Abrams

Cindy never planned to become a nurse; she was headed for a promising career in retail. Then her grandmother told her she had to become a nurse because she never wanted to go to a nursing home! Now, thirty-plus years later, Cindy enjoys being a champion for quality senior care. In addition to owning an assisted living home, Cindy's company provides care management and other services to the elderly and their families. She is very passionate about ensuring that seniors receive quality care, not only in the assisted living arena but in nursing homes and hospitals as well. Toward this end, she provides educational presentations to the public and professionals on important topics for the elderly and serves as a nurse advocate for her clients.

Index

A

abuse and neglect, 25, 64–65. *See also* Adult Protective Services (APS)
  legal responsibilities, 65
  signs of, 64–65
accusations. *See* abuse and neglect, signs of
activities. *See also* resident, individual preferences
  expectations about, 53
  individual preferences, 55
  and size of assisted living center, 61, 62–63
  state regulations about, 54
  types of, and relation to cost, 54–55
activities of daily living (ADLs), 9, 20. *See also* decline, signs of; personal care services
  that facilities are required to provide, 62
  and long-term care insurance, 24
  and service plans, 63
activity calendar, 54
Adult Protective Services (APS), 25, 65. *See also* resources, state and private; abuse and neglect, signs of
advance directives, 11, 58–60. *See also* orange cards; *Five Wishes, The*
advance planning, importance of, xiii–xiv
advanced life-support measures, 59. *See also* communication, importance of, with loved one